Ketogenic Slow Cooker Cookbook For Beginners

A Beginner's Guide With Quick And Easy Slow Cooker Recipes to Lose Weight For Your Keto Lifestyle

GW01057560

Tracy Flores

Disclaimer Notice:

Please note the information contained within this document is for educational and entertainment purposes only. All effort has been executed to present accurate, up to date, and reliable, complete information. No warranties of any kind are declared or implied. Readers acknowledge that the author is not engaging in the rendering of legal, financial, medical or professional advice. The content within this book has been derived from various sources. Please consult a licensed professional before attempting any techniques outlined in this book.

By reading this document, the reader agrees that under no circumstances is the author responsible for any losses, direct or indirect, which are incurred as a result of the use of information contained within this document, including, but not limited to, errors, omissions, or inaccuracies.

Table of Contents

Table of Content

Introduction

Thank you for purchasing **Ketogenic Slow Cooker Cookbook For Beginners: A Beginner's Guide With Quick And Easy Slow Cooker Recipes to Lose Weight For Your Keto Lifestyle**

It is called slow stove and it is one of the little great revolutions of contemporary cooking. To understand what it is, it is enough to understand its purpose, that is to cook food at low temperature, keeping almost unchanged their properties, but also rediscovering the good and healthy slow cooking of the past in the classic slow cooker.

The slow cooker, however, with respect to the latter, is an electrical instrument of a certain importance, composed by a base with wire and plug, a body which can have display, keyboards or simple knobs and a container (usually made of ceramic) where to put the food to be cooked. On the market it is possible to find different sizes and capacities, usually from 4 to 7 liters.

As said, slow cooking at low temperatures has the double function of not dispersing the vitamin properties of foods, as it happens instead when reaching and exceeding 100° C (212° F), but also to realize in a more practical way the classic traditional recipes. Those that actually require long preparations.

Stews, braises and stews are certainly enhanced by the use of the slow cooker, but you can also use it for less slow recipes, such as sauces, vegetable side dishes and even desserts. In this case the first candidates are creams, which, thanks to the low temperatures, will avoid sticking to the bottom of the container.

Breakfasts Recipes

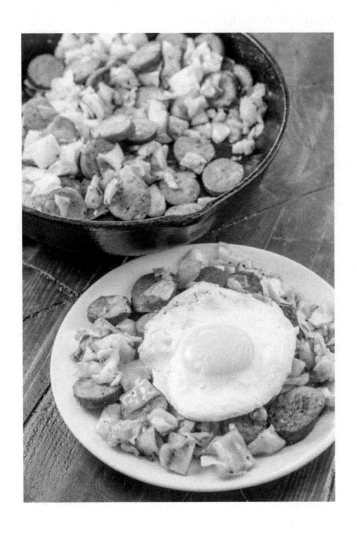

Healthy Low Carb Walnut Zucchini Bread

Preparation Time: 17 minutes

Cooking time: 3 hours 10 minutes

Servings: 12

Ingredients:

- 3 eggs

- 1/2 cup walnuts, chopped

- 2 cups zucchini, shredded

- 2 tsp vanilla

- 1/2 cup pure all-purpose sweetener

- 1/3 cup coconut oil, softened

- 1/2 tsp baking soda

- 1 1/2 Tsp baking powder

- 2 tsp cinnamon

- 1/3 cup coconut flour

- 1 cup almond flour

- 1/2 Tsp salt

Directions:

1.   In a bowl, combine almond flour, baking soda, baking powder, cinnamon, coconut flour, and salt. Set aside.

2.   In another bowl, whisk together eggs, vanilla, sweetener, and oil.

3.   Add dry mixture to the wet mixture and fold well.

4.   Add walnut and zucchini and fold well.

5.   Pour batter into the silicone bread pan.

6.   Place bread pan into the slow cooker on the rack.

7.   Cover slow cooker with lid and cook on high for 3 hours.

8.   Cut bread loaf into slices and serve.

Nutrition: calories 174, fat 15, carbs 5, protein 7

Savory Creamy Breakfast Casserole

Preparation Time: 17 minutes

Cooking time: 5 hours on low / 3 hours on high

Servings: 5

Ingredients:

• 1 tablespoon unsalted butter, Ghee (here), or extra-virgin olive oil

• 10 large eggs, beaten

• 1 cup heavy (whipping) cream

• 1½ cups shredded sharp Cheddar cheese, divided

• ½ cup grated Romano cheese

• ½ teaspoon kosher salt

• ¼ teaspoon freshly ground black pepper

• 8 ounces thick-cut ham, diced

• ¾ head broccoli, cut into small florets

• ½ onion, diced

Directions:

1. Generously coat the inside of the slow cooker insert with the butter.

2.   Directly in the insert, whisk together the eggs, heavy cream, ½ cup of Cheddar cheese, the Romano cheese, salt, and pepper.

3.   Stir in the ham, broccoli, and onion.

4.   Sprinkle the remaining 1 cup of Cheddar cheese over the top. Cover and cook for 6 hours on low or 3 hours on high. Serve hot.

Nutrition: calories 465, fat 10, carbs 7, protein 28

Breakfast Cauliflower Hash

Preparation Time: 17 minutes

Cooking time: 8 hours

Servings: 5

Ingredients:

- 7 eggs

- ¼ cup milk

- 1 teaspoon salt

- 1 teaspoon ground black pepper

- ½ teaspoon ground mustard

- 10 oz. cauliflower

- ¼ teaspoon chili flakes

- 5 oz. breakfast sausages, chopped

- ½ onion, chopped

- 5 oz. Cheddar cheese, shredded

Directions:

1. Wash the cauliflower carefully and separate it into the florets.

2. After this, shred the cauliflower florets.

3.   Beat the eggs in a bowl and whisk. Add the milk, salt, ground black pepper, ground mustard, chili flakes, and chopped onion into the whisked egg mixture.

4.   Put the shredded cauliflower in the slow cooker.

5.   Add the whisked egg mixture. Add the shredded cheese and chopped sausages.

6.   Stir the mixture gently and close the slow cooker lid.

7.   Cook the dish on LOW for 8 hours. When the cauliflower hash is cooked, remove it from the slow cooker and mix up. Enjoy!

Nutrition: calories 329, fat 16, carbs 10, protein 23

Breakfast Sweet Pepper Rounds

Preparation Time: 10 minutes

Cooking time: 3 hours

Servings: 4

Ingredients:

- 2 red sweet pepper

- 7 oz. ground chicken

- 5 oz. Parmesan

- 1 tablespoon sour cream

- 1 tablespoon flour

- 1 egg

- 2 teaspoon almond milk

- 1 teaspoon salt

- ½ teaspoon ground black pepper

- ¼ teaspoon butter

Directions:

1.   Combine the sour cream with the ground chicken, flour, ground black pepper, almond milk, and butter.

2.   Beat eggs into the mixture.

3. Remove the seeds from the sweet peppers and slice them roughly.

4. Place the pepper slices in the slow cooker and fill them with the ground chicken mixture.

5. After this, chop Parmesan into the cubes and add them to the sliced peppers.

6. Close the slow cooker lid and cook the dish for 3 hours on HIGH.

7. When the time is done make sure that the ground chicken is cooked and the cheese is melted. Enjoy the dish immediately.

Nutrition: calories 261, fat 8, carbs 13, protein 21

Lunch Recipes

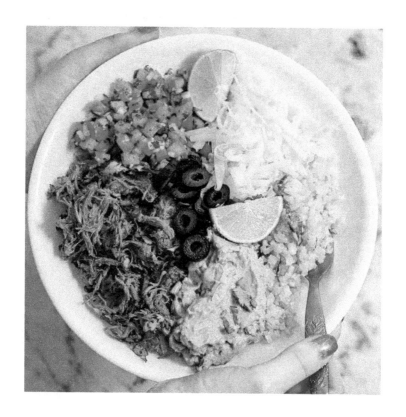

Tuna in Potatoes

Preparation time: 16 minutes

Cooking time: 4 hours

Servings: 8

Ingredients:

- 4 large potatoes

- 8 oz. tuna, canned

- ½ cup cream cheese

- 4 oz. Cheddar cheese

- 1 garlic clove

- 1 teaspoon onion powder

- ½ teaspoon salt

- 1 teaspoon ground black pepper

- 1 teaspoon dried dill

Directions:

1.   Wash the potatoes carefully and cut them into the halves.

2.   Wrap the potatoes in the foil and place in the slow cooker. Close the slow cooker lid and cook the potatoes on HIGH for 2 hours.

3.   Meanwhile, peel the garlic clove and mince it. Combine the minced garlic clove with the cream cheese, tuna, salt, ground black pepper, onion powder, and dill.

4.   Then shred Cheddar cheese and add it to the mixture.

5.   Mix it carefully until homogenous.

6.   When the time is over – remove the potatoes from the slow cooker and discard the foil only from the flat surface of the potatoes.

7.   Then take the fork and mash the flesh of the potato halves gently. Add the tuna mixture in the potato halves and return them back in the slow cooker.

8.   Cook the potatoes for 2 hours more on HIGH. Enjoy!

Nutrition:

Calories 247,

Fat 5.9,

Fiber 4,

Carbs 35.31,

Protein 14

Sweet Corn Pilaf

Preparation time: 21 minutes

Cooking time: 8 hours

Servings: 5

Ingredients:

- 2 cups rice

- 1 cup sweet corn, frozen

- 6 oz. chicken fillet

- 1 sweet red pepper

- 1 yellow sweet pepper

- ½ cup green peas, frozen

- 1 carrot

- 4 cups chicken stock

- 2 tablespoon chopped almonds

- 1 teaspoon olive oil

- 1 teaspoon salt

- 1 teaspoon ground white pepper

Directions:

1. Peel the carrot and cut into the small cubes.

2.   Combine the carrot cubes with the frozen sweet corn and green peas.

3.   After this, place the vegetable mixture in the slow cooker vessel.

4.   Add the rice, chicken stock, olive oil, salt, and ground white pepper.

5.   After this, cut the chicken fillet into the strips and add the meat to the rice mixture.

6.   Chop all the sweet peppers and add them in the slow cooker too.

7.   Close the slow cooker lid and cook the pilaf for 8 hours on LOW.

8.   When the pilaf is cooked, stir it gently and sprinkle with the almonds. Mix the dish carefully again. Serve it immediately. Enjoy!

Nutrition:

Calories 390,

Fat 18.6,

Fiber 13,

Carbs 54.7,

Banana Lunch Sandwiches

Preparation time: 15 minutes

Cooking time: 2 hours

Servings: 4

Ingredients:

- 2 banana

- 8 oz. French toast slices, frozen

- 1 tablespoon peanut butter

- ¼ teaspoon ground cinnamon

- 5 oz. Cheddar cheese, sliced

- ¼ teaspoon turmeric

Directions:

1. Peel the bananas and slice them.

2. Spread the French toast slices with the peanut butter well. Combine the ground cinnamon with the turmeric and stir the mixture. Sprinkle the French toasts with the spice mixture.

3. Then make the layer of the sliced bananas on the toasts and add the sliced cheese.

4. Cover the toast with the second part of the toast to make the sandwich.

5.   Place the banana sandwiches in the slow cooker and cook them on HIGH for 2 hours.

6.   Serve the prepared banana sandwiches hot. Enjoy!

Nutrition:

Calories 248,

Fat 7.5,

Fiber 2,

Carbs 36.74,

Protein 10

Chicken Open Sandwich

Preparation time: 15 minutes

Cooking time: 8 hours

Servings: 4

Ingredients:

- 7 oz. chicken fillet
- 1 teaspoon cayenne pepper
- 5 oz. mashed potato, cooked
- 6 tablespoons chicken gravy
- 4 slices French bread, toasted
- 2 teaspoons mayo
- 1 cup water

Directions:

1. Put the chicken fillet in the slow cooker and sprinkle it with the cayenne pepper.

2. Add water and chicken gravy. Close the slow cooker lid and cook the chicken for 8 hours on LOW. Then combine the mashed potato with the mayo sauce.

3. Spread toasted French bread with the mashed potato mixture.

4.   When the chicken is cooked, cut it into the strips and combine with the remaining gravy from the slow cooker.

5.   Place the chicken strips over the mashed potato. Enjoy the open sandwich warm!

Nutrition:

Calories 314,

Fat 9.7,

Fiber 3,

Carbs 45.01,

Protein 12

Light Lunch Quiche

Preparation time: 21 minutes

Cooking time: 4 hours 25 minutes

Servings: 7

Ingredients:

- 7 oz. pie crust
- ¼ cup broccoli
- 1/3 cup sweet peas
- ¼ cup heavy cream
- 2 tablespoons flour
- 3 eggs
- 4 oz. Romano cheese, shredded
- 1 teaspoon cilantro
- 1 teaspoon salt
- ¼ cup spinach
- 1 tomato

Directions:

1. Cover the inside of the slow cooker bowl with parchment.

2.   Put the pie crust inside and flatten it well with your fingertips.

3.   Chop the broccoli and combine it with sweet peas. Combine the heavy cream, flour, cilantro, and salt together. Stir the liquid until smooth.

4.   Then beat the eggs into the heavy cream liquid and mix it with a hand mixer. When you get a smooth mix, combine it with the broccoli.

5.   Chop the spinach and add it to the mix. Chop the tomato and add it to the mix too. Pour the prepared mixture into the pie crust slowly.

6.   Close the slow cooker lid and cook the quiche for 4 hours on HIGH.

7.   After 4 hours, sprinkle the quiche surface with the shredded cheese and cook the dish for 25 minutes more. Serve the prepared quiche! Enjoy!

Nutrition:

Calories 287,

Fat 18.8,

Fiber 1,

Carbs 17.1,

Protein 11

Dinner Recipes

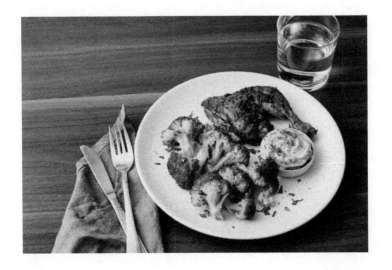

Sautéed Greens

Preparation time: 15 minutes

Cooking time: 1 hour

Servings: 4

Ingredients:

- 1 cup spinach, chopped

- 2 cups collard greens, chopped

- 1 cup Swiss chard, chopped

- water

- ½ cup half and half

Directions

Put spinach, collard greens, and Swiss chard in the slow cooker.

Add water and close the lid.

Cook the greens on High for 1 hour.

Then drain water and transfer the greens in the bowl.

Bring the half and half to boil and pour over greens.

Carefully mix the greens.

Nutrition 49 calories, 1.8g protein, 3.2g carbohydrates, 3.7g fat, 1.1g fiber, 11mg cholesterol, 45mg sodium, 117mg potassium.

Duck Breast

Preparation time: 10 minutes Cooking time: 5 hours

Servings: 4

Ingredients:

- 1 teaspoon liquid stevia

- 1-pound duck breast, boneless, skinless

- 1 teaspoon chili pepper

- 2 tablespoons butter

- ½ cup water

- 1 bay leaf

Directions:

Rub the duck breast with the chili pepper and liquid stevia, then transfer it to the slow cooker.

Add the bay leaf and water.

Add butter and close the lid. Cook the duck breast for 5 hours on Low.

Let the cooked duck breast rest for 10 minutes, then remove it from the slow cooker. Slice it into the servings. Enjoy!

Nutrition: calories 199 fat 10.3, fiber 0.1, carbs 0.3, protein 25.1

Potato Salad

Preparation time: 10 minutes

Cooking time: 3 hours

Servings: 2

Ingredients:

- 1 cup potato, chopped
- 1 cup of water
- 1 teaspoon salt
- oz. celery stalk, chopped
- oz. fresh parsley, chopped
- ¼ onion, diced
- 1 tablespoon mayonnaise

Directions

Put the potatoes in the slow cooker. Add water and salt. Cook the potatoes on High for 3 hours. Then drain water and transfer the potatoes in the salad bowl. Add all remaining ingredients and carefully mix the salad.

Nutrition 129 calories, 5.5g protein, 12.4g carbohydrates, 6.7g fat, 2.5g fiber, 12mg cholesterol, 1479mg sodium, 465mg potassium.

Lamb Chops

Preparation time: 15 minutes Cooking time: 3 hours Servings: 2

Ingredients:

- oz lamb chops
- 1 tablespoon tomato puree
- ½ teaspoon cumin
- ½ teaspoon ground coriander
- 1 teaspoon garlic powder
- 1 teaspoon butter
- tablespoons water

Directions:

Mix the tomato puree, cumin, ground coriander, garlic powder, and water in the bowl. Brush the lamb chops with the tomato puree mixture on each side and let marinate for 20 minutes. Toss the butter in the slow cooker. Add the lamb chops and close the lid.

Cook the lamb chops for 3 hours on High.

Transfer the cooked lamb onto serving plates and enjoy!

Nutrition: calories 290, fat 12.5, fiber 0.4, carbs 2, protein 40.3

Ropa Vieja

Preparation Time: 15 minutes

Cooking Time: 8 hours

Servings: 6

Ingredients:

- 2 lb. flank steak – remove fat

1 of each:

- Yellow pepper

- Thinly sliced onion

- Green pepper

- Bay leaf

- ¼ t. salt

¾ t. of each:

- Oregano

- Non-fat beef broth

- Tomato paste

- Cooking spray

Directions:

Prepare the slow cooker with the spray or use a liner and combine all of the fixings.

Stir everything together and prepare using low for eight hours.

Top it off with your chosen garnishes.

Nutrition:

Calories: 257

Net Carbs: 7 g

Fat: 10 g

Protein: 35 g

Spinach Soup

Preparation Time: 15 minutes

Cooking Time: 6-8 hours

Servings: 4

Ingredients:

- 2 pounds spinach

- ¼ cup cream cheese

- 1 onion, diced

- 2 cups heavy cream

- 1 garlic clove, minced

- 2 cups water

- salt, pepper, to taste

Directions:

Pour water into the slow cooker. Add spinach, salt, and pepper.

Add cream cheese, onion, garlic, and heavy cream.

Close the lid and cook on Low for 6-8 hours.

Puree soup with blender and serve.

Nutrition: Calories 322 Fats 28.2g Net carbs 10.1g Protein 12.2g

Jerk Chicken

Preparation time: 25 minutes

Cooking time: 5 hours

Servings: 4

Ingredients:

- 1 teaspoon nutmeg

- 1 teaspoon cinnamon

- 1 teaspoon minced garlic

- ½ teaspoon cloves

- 1 teaspoon ground coriander

- 1 tablespoon Erythritol

- 1-pound chicken thighs

- ½ cup water

- 1 tablespoon butter

Directions:

Mix the nutmeg, cinnamon, minced garlic, cloves, and ground coriander.

Add Erythritol and stir the ingredients until well blended.

Sprinkle the chicken thighs with the spice mixture.

Let the chicken thighs sit for 10 minutes to marinate, then put the chicken thighs in the slow cooker.

Add the butter and water.

Close the lid and cook Jerk chicken for 5 hours on Low.

Serve Jerk chicken immediately!

Nutrition:

calories 247,

fat 11.5,

fiber 0.5,

carbs 4.9,

protein 33

Main

Pork Shoulder

Preparation time: 25 minutes

Cooking time: 7 hours

Servings: 6

Ingredients:

- 1-pound pork shoulder

- 2 cups water

- 1 onion, peeled

- 2 garlic cloves, peeled

- 1 teaspoon peppercorns

- 1 teaspoon chili flakes

- ½ teaspoon paprika

- 1 teaspoon turmeric

- 1 teaspoon cumin

Directions:

Sprinkle the pork shoulder with the peppercorns, chili flakes, paprika, turmeric, and cumin.

Stir it well and let it sit for 15 minutes to marinate.

Transfer the pork shoulder to the slow cooker.

Add water and peeled the onion.

Add garlic cloves and close the lid.

Cook the pork shoulder for 7 hours on Low.

Remove the pork shoulder from the slow cooker and serve!

Nutrition:

calories 234,

fat 16.4,

fiber 0.7,

carbs 2.8,

protein 18

Soups, Stews, and Chilis

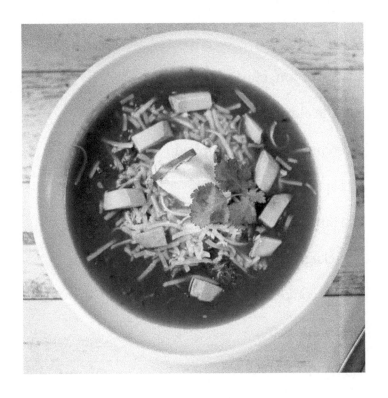

Beans and Squash Chili

Preparation Time: 10 minutes

Cooking time: 8 Hours 15 Minutes

Servings: 6

Ingredients:

- 1 tbsp. olive oil

- 1 large onion, chopped

- 1 garlic clove, minced

- 3 red bell peppers, chopped

- 2 tbsp. chili powder

- 1/2 tsp. ground cumin

- 2 packages (12 oz.) cubed butternut squash

- 3 cups cooked pinto beans

- 1 1/2 cups water

- 1 1/2 cups water

- 1 cup frozen whole-kernel corn

- 1 tsp. salt

- 1 can (14 1/2 oz.) chopped green chilies, undrained

- 3/4 queso fresco or feta, crumbled

- Lime wedges

Directions:

1. Heat the oil in a skillet. Sauté the onion, garlic, and bell pepper.

2. Season with chili and cumin while sautéing. Transfer to a slow cooker.

3. Add the squash, pinto beans, water, corn, salt, tomatoes, and chilies.

4. Cover and cook for 8 hours on LOW. Vegetables should be tender and soup should be thick.

5. Serve topped with cheese and lime. Enjoy!

Nutrition: calories 316, fat 2, carbs 10, protein 18

Tasty Beef Thyme Pot Roast

Preparation Time: 15 minutes

Cooking time: 7 hours

Servings: 4

Ingredients:

- 3 pounds of beef chuck roast
- 2 tablespoons of olive oil
- 1 red onion sliced into tiny pieces
- 2 cups of hot water
- 1 cup of beef broth
- 2 tablespoons of butter
- 1 teaspoon of dried rosemary
- 1 teaspoon of dried thyme
- Salt and pepper
- 5 small turnips peeled and cut into strips

Directions:

1. Heat the olive oil in a frying pan over high heat and brown the meat on both sides for 2 minutes.

2. Place all ingredients except the turnips into the slow cooker.

3. Cover and cook for five hours on low.

4. Add the turnips and cook for a further 2 hours until the turnips soften.

5. Spoon onto dishes and serve with garlic sauce or sour cream.

Nutrition: calories 231, fat 16, carbs 13, protein 28

Butternut Squash Soup with Parsnips

Preparation Time: 10 minutes

Cooking time: 6 Hours 10 Minutes

Servings: 8

Ingredients:

- 1 large sweet onion, chopped

- 3 large parsnips, peeled and chopped

- 1 large Granny Smith apple, peeled and chopped

- 1/4 tsp. salt

- 1 tsp. freshly ground black pepper

- 3 cups water

- 2 cups chicken broth, low-sodium, fat-free

- 3 packages (12 oz.) frozen butternut squash, thawed

- 2 tbsp. whipping cream or coconut cream

- 1/8 tsp. paprika

- 1/8 tsp. ground cumin

- 1/2 cup light sour cream

- Chopped fresh chives (optional)

Directions:

1.   Place the onion, parsnips, apple, salt, pepper, water, broth, and squash in the slow cooker. Stir.

2.   Cover and cook for 6 hours on LOW.

3.   Puree using an immersion blender until smooth. (A regular blender may also be used. Puree in small batches to prevent spillage. Be careful, liquid is hot! Remove lid insert to allow steam to escape.)

4.   Stir in the whipping cream, paprika, and cumin.

5.   Serve with a dollop of sour cream on top, sprinkled with chives. Enjoy!

Nutrition: calories 131, fat 5, carbs 13, protein 4

Fish and Seafood

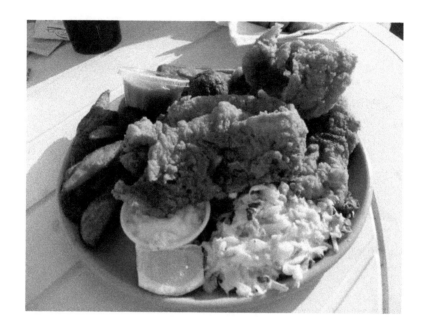

Creamy Tuna

Preparation Time: 10 minutes

Cooking time: 4 hours

Servings: 6

Ingredients:

- 1-pound tuna fillet, boneless and cubed

- 1 red chili pepper, minced

- 1 tablespoon butter

- 2 shallots, chopped

- ½ cup heavy cream

- 1 cup Mozzarella cheese, shredded

- 1 teaspoon salt

- 1 teaspoon paprika

- 1 teaspoon basil, dried

Directions:

1.   Put butter in the bottom of the slow cooker.

2.   Add the tuna and the other ingredients and toss.

3.   Close the lid and cook for 4 hours on High.

Nutrition: calories 205, fat 12, carbs 9, protein 21

Italian Shrimp Tortillas

Preparation Time: 10 minutes

Cooking time: 2 hours

Servings: 2

Ingredients:

- 2 keto tortillas

- ½ teaspoon Cajun seasoning

- 1 teaspoon Italian seasoning

- 1 tablespoon chives, chopped

- 2 tablespoons fresh cilantro, chopped

- 2 oz Cheddar cheese, shredded

- 7 oz shrimps, peeled

- ½ cup heavy cream

- ½ teaspoon ground coriander

- 1 teaspoon salt

- 1 jalapeno pepper, sliced

Directions:

1.   In the slow cooker, mix the shrimp with the seasonings and the other ingredients and close the lid. Cook shrimps on High for 2 hours.

2.   After this, fill keto tortillas with shrimps and serve.

Nutrition: calories 220, fat 6, carbs 5, protein 6

Salmon and Radish Soup

Preparation Time: 10 minutes

Cooking time: 3 hours

Servings: 4

Ingredients:

- 1 cup radishes, halved
- 10 oz salmon, chopped
- 1 teaspoon lime juice
- 1 teaspoon lime zest, grated
- ½ cup of coconut milk
- 2 cups of water
- 1 teaspoon salt
- 1 teaspoon garlic, diced
- ½ teaspoon chives, chopped

Directions:

1. In the slow cooker, mix the salmon with radishes and the other ingredients.

2. Close the lid and cook the liquid for 2.5 hours on High.

3. Divide into bowls and serve.

Nutrition: calories 214, fat 5, carbs 7, protein 9

Vegetables

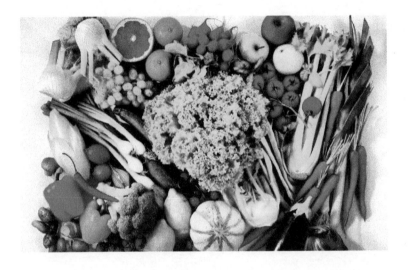

Zucchini Mix

Preparation time: 10 minutes

Cooking time: 3 hours

Servings: 6

Ingredients

- 1-pound zucchinis, roughly cubed

- 2 spring onions, chopped

- 1 teaspoon curry paste

- 1 teaspoon basil, dried

- 1 teaspoon salt

- 1 teaspoon ground black pepper

- 1 bay leaf

- ½ cup beef stock

Directions:

1. In the slow cooker, mix the zucchinis with the onion and the other Ingredients.

2. Close the lid and cook on Low for 3 hours.

Nutrition: calories 34, fat 1.3, fiber 3.6, carbs 4.7, protein 3.6

Red Cabbage and Walnuts

Preparation time: 15 minutes

Cooking time: 6 hours

Servings: 4

Ingredients

- 2 cups red cabbage, shredded

- 3 spring onions, chopped

- ½ cup chicken stock

- 1 tablespoon olive oil

- 1 teaspoon salt

- 1 teaspoon cumin, ground

- 1 teaspoon hot paprika

- 1 tablespoon Keto tomato sauce

- 1 oz. walnuts

- 1/3 cup fresh parsley, chopped

Directions:

1. In the slow cooker, mix the cabbage with the spring onions and the other Ingredients.

2. Close the lid and cook cabbage for 6 hours on Low.

3. Divide into bowls and serve.

Nutrition: calories 112, fat 5.1, fiber 2, carbs 5.8, protein 3.5

Paprika Bok Choy

Preparation time: 15 minutes

Cooking time: 2.5 hours

Servings: 6

Ingredients

- 1-pound bok choy, torn
- ½ cup of coconut milk
- 1 tablespoon almond butter, softened
- 1 teaspoon ground paprika
- 1 teaspoon turmeric
- ½ teaspoon cayenne pepper

Directions:

1. In the slow cooker, mix the bok choy with the coconut milk and the other Ingredients, toss and close the lid.

2. Cook the meal for 2.5 hours on High.

Nutrition: calories 128, fat 3.2, fiber 3.9, carbs 4.9, protein 4.1

Spinach and Olives Mix

Preparation time: 15 minutes

Cooking time: 3.5 hours

Servings: 6

Ingredients

- 2 cups spinach

- 2 tablespoons chives, chopped

- 5 oz. Cheddar cheese, shredded

- ½ cup heavy cream

- 1 teaspoon ground black pepper

- ½ teaspoon salt

- 1 cup black olives, pitted and halved

- 1 teaspoon sage

- 1 teaspoon sweet paprika

Directions:

1.   In the slow cooker, mix the spinach with the chives and the other Ingredients, toss and close the lid.

2.   Cook for 3.5 hours on Low and serve.

Nutrition: calories 189, fat 6.2, fiber 0.6, carbs 3, protein 3.4

Zucchini and Spring Onions

Preparation time: 20 minutes

Cooking time: 2 hours

Servings: 8

Ingredients

- 1-pound zucchinis, sliced

- 1 teaspoon avocado oil

- 1 teaspoon salt

- 1 teaspoon white pepper

- 2 spring onions, chopped

- 1/3 cup organic almond milk

- 2 tablespoons butter

- ½ teaspoon turmeric powder

Directions:

1. In the slow cooker, mix the zucchinis with the spring onions, oil and the other Ingredients.

2. Close the lid and cook for 2 hours on High.

Nutrition: calories 82, fat 5.6, fiber 2.8, carbs 5.6, protein 3.2

Cauliflower and Turmeric Mash

Preparation time: 10 minutes

Cooking time: 3 hours

Servings: 3

Ingredients

- 1 cup cauliflower florets

- 1 teaspoon turmeric powder

- 1 cup of water

- 1 teaspoon salt

- 1 tablespoon butter

- 1 tablespoon coconut cream

- 1 teaspoon coriander, ground

Directions:

1.   In the slow cooker, mix the cauliflower with water and salt.

2.   Close the lid and cook for 3 hours on High.

3.   Then drain water and transfer the cauliflower to a blender.

4.   Add the rest of the Ingredients, blend and serve.

Nutrition: calories 58, fat 5.2, fiber 1.2, carbs 2.7, protein 1.1

Meat

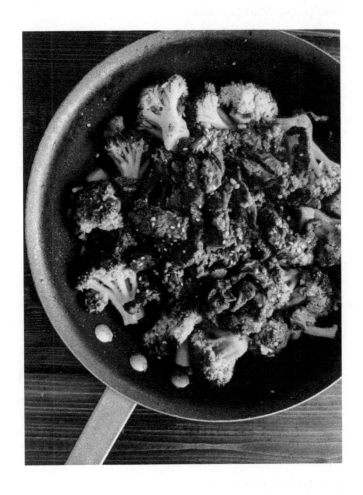

Beef and Scallions Bowl

Preparation time: 10 minutes Cooking time: 5 hours Servings: 4 Ingredients

- 1 teaspoon chili powder
- 2 oz. scallions, chopped
- 1-pound beef stew meat, cubed
- 1 cup corn kernels, frozen
- 1 cup of water
- 2 tablespoons tomato paste
- 1 teaspoon minced garlic

Directions

1   Mix water with tomato paste and pour the liquid into the slow cooker.

2   Add chili powder, beef, corn kernels, and minced garlic.

3   Close the lid and cook the meal on high for 5 hours.

4   When the meal is cooked, transfer the mixture to the bowls and top with scallions.

Nutrition : 258 calories, 36.4g protein, 0.4g carbohydrates, 7.7g fat, 2g fiber, 101mg cholesterol, 99mg sodium, 697mg potassium.

Beef with Greens

Preparation time: 15 minutes Cooking time: 8 hours

Servings: 3 Ingredients

- 1 cup fresh spinach, chopped

- oz. beef stew meat, cubed

- 1 cup Swiss chard, chopped

- 2 cups of water

- 1 teaspoon olive oil

- 1 teaspoon dried rosemary

Directions

1   Heat olive oil in the skillet.

2   Add beef and roast it for 1 minute per side.

3   Then transfer the meat to the slow cooker.

4   Add Swiss chard, spinach, water, and rosemary.

5   Close the lid and cook the meal on Low for 8 hours.

Nutrition : 177 calories, 26.3g protein, 1.1g carbohydrates, 7g fat, 0.6g fiber, 76mg cholesterol, 95mg sodium, 449mg potassium.

Chili Lime Beef

Preparation time: 10 minutes Cooking time: 6 hours

Servings: 4

Ingredients

- 1 lb. beef chuck roast
- 1 tsp chili powder
- 2 cups lemon-lime soda
- 1 fresh lime juice
- 1 garlic clove, crushed
- 1/2 tsp salt

Directions:

- Place beef chuck roast into the slow cooker.
- Season roast with garlic, chili powder, and salt.
- Pour lemon-lime soda over the roast.
- Cover slow cooker with lid and cook on low for 6 hours.

Shred the meat using a fork.

- Add lime juice over shredded roast and serve.

Nutrition: Calories 355 Fat 16.8 g Carbohydrates 14 g Sugar 11.3 g Protein 35.5 g Cholesterol 120 mg

Beefin Sauce

Preparation time: 10 minutes Cooking time: 9 hours

Servings: 4 Ingredients

- 1-pound beef stew meat, chopped

- 1 teaspoon gram masala

- 1 cup of water

- 1 tablespoon flour

- 1 teaspoon garlic powder

- 1 onion, diced

Directions

1   Whisk flour with water until smooth and pour the liquid into the slow cooker.

2   Add gram masala and beef stew meat. After this, add onion and garlic powder. Close the lid and cook the meat on low for 9 hours.

3   Serve the cooked beef with thick gravy from the slow cooker.

Nutrition : 231 calories, 35g protein, 4.6g carbohydrates, 7.1g fat, 0.7g fiber, 101mg cholesterol, 79mg sodium, 507mg potassium

Beef Stroganoff

Preparation time: 10 minutes

Cooking time: 8 hours

Servings: 2

Ingredients

- 1/2 lb. beef stew meat

- 1/2 cup sour cream

- 2.5 oz. mushrooms, sliced

- oz. mushroom soup

- 1 medium onion, chopped

- Pepper and salt

Directions:

- Add all Ingredients: except sour cream into the slow cooker and mix well. Cover slow cooker with lid and cook on low for 8 hours. Add sour cream and stir well. Serve and enjoy.

Nutrition:

Calories 471 Fat 25.3 g Carbohydrates 8.6 g Sugar 3.1 g Protein 48.9 g

Cholesterol 109 mg

Side Dish Recipes

Lemony Pumpkin Wedges

Preparation time: 15 minutes

Cooking time: 6 Hours

Servings: 4

Ingredients

- 15 oz. pumpkin, peeled and cut into wedges
- 1 tbsp. lemon juice
- 1 tsp. salt
- 1 tsp. honey
- ½ tsp. ground cardamom
- 1 tsp. lime juice

Directions:

1. Add pumpkin, lemon juice, honey, lime juice, cardamom, and salt to the Crock Pot.

2. Put the slow cooker's lid on and set the cooking time to 6 hours on Low settings.

3. Serve fresh.

Nutrition: Per Serving: Calories: 35, Total Fat: 0.1g, Fiber: 1g, Total Carbs: 8.91g, Protein: 1g

Eggplants with Mayo Sauce

Preparation time: 15 minutes

Cooking time: 5 Hours

Servings: 8

Ingredients

- 2 tbsp. minced garlic
- 1 chili pepper, chopped
- 1 sweet pepper, chopped
- 4 tbsp. mayo
- 1 tsp. olive oil
- 1 tsp. salt
- ½ tsp. ground black pepper
- 18 oz. eggplants, peeled and diced
- 2 tbsp. sour cream

Directions:

1. Blend chili pepper, sweet peppers, salt, garlic, and black pepper in a blender until smooth.

2. Add eggplant and this chili mixture to the Crock Pot then toss them well.

3.   Now mix mayo with sour cream and spread on top of eggplants.

4.   Put the cooker's lid on and set the cooking time to 5 hours on High settings.

5.   Serve warm

Nutrition: Per Serving: Calories: 40, Total Fat: 1.1g, Fiber: 3g, Total Carbs: 7.5g, Protein: 1g

Summer Squash Medley

Preparation time: 15 minutes

Cooking time: 2 hours

Servings: 4

Ingredients

- ¼ cup olive oil
- 2 tbsp. basil, chopped
- 2 tbsp. balsamic vinegar
- 2 garlic cloves, minced
- 2 tsp. mustard
- Salt and black pepper to the taste
- 3 summer squash, sliced
- 2 zucchinis, sliced

Directions:

1. Add squash, zucchinis, and all other Ingredients: to the Crock Pot.

2. Put the cooker's lid on and set the cooking time to hours on High settings.

3. Serve.

Nutrition: Per Serving: Calories: 179, Total Fat: 13g, Fiber: 2g, Total Carbs: 10g, Protein: 4g

Broccoli Mix

Preparation time: 15 minutes

Cooking time: 2 Hours

Servings: 10

Ingredients

- 6 cups broccoli florets
- 1 and ½ cups cheddar cheese, shredded
- 10 ounces canned cream of celery soup
- ½ teaspoon Worcestershire sauce
- ¼ cup yellow onion, chopped
- Salt and black pepper to the taste
- 1 cup crackers, crushed
- 2 tablespoons soft butter

Directions:

1.   In a bowl, mix broccoli with cream of celery soup, cheese, salt, pepper, onion and Worcestershire sauce, toss and transfer to your Crock Pot.

2.   Add butter, toss again, sprinkle crackers, cover and cook on High for hours.

3.   Serve as a side dish.

Nutrition: calories 159, fat 11, fiber 1, carbs 11, protein 6

Roasted Beets

Preparation time: 15 minutes

Cooking time: 4 Hours

Servings: 5

Ingredients

- 10 small beets

- 5 teaspoons olive oil

- A pinch of salt and black pepper

Directions:

1.   Divide each beet on a tin foil piece, drizzle oil, season them with salt and pepper, rub well, wrap beets, place them in your Crock Pot, cover and cook on High for 4 hours.

2.   Unwrap beets, cool them down a bit, peel, and slice and serve them as a side dish.

Nutrition: calories 100, fat 2, fiber 2, carbs 4, protein 5

Thai Side Salad

Preparation time: 15 minutes

Cooking time: 3 Hours

Servings: 8

Ingredients

•   8 ounces yellow summer squash, peeled and roughly chopped

•   12 ounces zucchini, halved and sliced

•   2 cups button mushrooms, quartered

•   1 red sweet potatoes, chopped

•   2 leeks, sliced

•   2 tablespoons veggie stock

•   2 garlic cloves, minced

•   2 tablespoon Thai red curry paste

•   1 tablespoon ginger, grated

•   1/3 cup coconut milk

•   ¼ cup basil, chopped

Directions:

1.   In your Crock Pot, mix zucchini with summer squash, mushrooms, red pepper, leeks, garlic, stock, curry paste,

ginger, coconut milk and basil, toss, cover and cook on Low for

3 hours.

2. Stir your Thai mix one more time, divide between

plates and serve as a side dish.

Nutrition: calories 69, fat 2, fiber 2, carbs 8, protein 2

Appetizers & Snacks

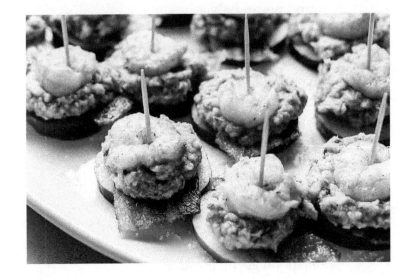

Flavorful Pecans

Preparation time: 15 minutes

Cooking time: 2 hours & 30 minutes

Servings: 16

Ingredients

- 1-pound pecan halves

- ¼ cup butter, melted

- 1 teaspoon dried oregano

- 1 teaspoon dried basil

- 1 teaspoon dried thyme

- 1 tablespoon red chili powder

- ½ teaspoon onion powder

- ¼ teaspoon garlic powder

- ¼ teaspoon cayenne pepper

- Salt, to taste

Directions:

1   Combine all fixings in a large slow cooker.

2   Cook in the slow cooker on high and cook, covered, for about 15 minutes.

3   Uncover the slow cooker and stir the mixture.

4   Cook on low, uncovered, within 2 hours, mixing occasionally.

5   Transfer the pecans into a bowl and keep aside to cool before serving.

Nutrition:

Calories: 225

Carbohydrates: 4.5g

Protein: 3.2g

Fat: 23.2g

Sugar: 1.1g

Sodium: 37mg

Fiber: 3.3g

Herb Flavored Almonds

Preparation time: 15 minutes

Cooking time: 2 hours

Servings: 16

Ingredients

- 2 cups of raw almonds

- 1 tablespoon olive oil

- 1 tablespoon dried rosemary

- 1 tablespoon dried thyme

- Salt

- ground black pepper

Directions:

1   Mix all the fixings in a large slow cooker.

2   Cook in the slow cooker on high and cook, covered, for about 1½ hours, stirring after every 30 minutes. Cool before serving.

Nutrition:Calories: 77 Carbohydrates: 2.8g Protein: 2.5g Fat: 6.9g Sugar: 0.5g Sodium: 12mg Fiber: 1.6g

Zesty Chicken Wings

Preparation time: 15 minutes

Cooking time: 7 hours & 12 minutes

Servings: 8

Ingredients

- For Sauce:

- ¼ cup low-sodium soy sauce

- ¼ cup fresh lime juice

- tablespoons Erythritol

- 1 teaspoon Sriracha

- 1 teaspoon ginger powder

- 2 garlic cloves, minced

- 1 teaspoon fresh lime zest, grated finely

- For Wings:

- 2 pounds grass-fed chicken wings

- teaspoons arrowroot starch

- 1 tablespoon water

Directions:

1   For the sauce: Put all sauce fixings in a large bowl, and beat until well combined.

2   Put chicken wings at the bottom of a slow cooker, and top with sauce evenly.

3   Set on low setting and cook, covered, for about 6-7 hours.

4   Dissolve arrowroot starch in water in a small bowl.

5   Uncover the slow cooker and stir in arrowroot mixture until well combined.

6   Cook on high, covered, for about 10-12 minutes.

7   Serve immediately.

Nutrition:

Calories: 456 Carbohydrates: 12.6g

Protein: 66.8g Fat: 16.9g

Sugar: 8.6g Sodium: 1084mg

Fiber: 0.2g

Candied Walnuts

Preparation time: 15 minutes

Cooking time: 2 hours & 30 minutes

Servings: 16

Ingredients

*   ½ cup unsalted butter

*   1-pound walnuts

*   ½ cup Splenda, granular

*   1½ teaspoons ground cinnamon

*   ¼ teaspoon ground allspice

*   ¼ teaspoon ground ginger

*   1/8 teaspoon ground cloves

Directions:

1   Set a slow cooker on high and preheat for about 15 minutes. Add butter and walnuts and stir to combine.

2   Add the Splenda and stir to combine well. Cook, covered, for about 15 minutes.

3   Uncover the slow cooker and stir the mixture. Set to cook on low, uncovered, within 2 hours, stirring occasionally.

4   Transfer the walnuts to a bowl. In another small bowl, mix spices.

5   Sift spice mixture over walnuts and toss to coat evenly. Set aside to cool before serving.

Nutrition:

Calories: 227

Carbohydrates: 10.5g

Protein: 6.9g

Fat: 22.5g

Sugar: 7g

Sodium: 42mg

Fiber: 2.1g

Tastier Nuts Combo

Preparation time: 15 minutes

Cooking time: 2 hours

Servings: 32

Ingredients

- 1 cup hazelnuts, toasted and skins removed

- 1 cup whole almonds, toasted

- 1 cup pecan halves, toasted

- 1 cup whole cashews

- ½ cup Erythritol

- 1/3 cup butter, melted

- ½ teaspoon ground cinnamon

- ½ teaspoon ground ginger

- ¼ teaspoon ground cloves

- ¼ teaspoon cayenne pepper

Directions:

1   In a large slow cooker, add all fixings and stir to combine.

2   Set on low, covered, cook for about 2 hours, stirring once after 1 hour.

3   Uncover the slow cooker and stir nuts again.

4   Transfer nuts onto a sheet of buttered foil to cool for at least 1 hour before serving.

Nutrition:

Calories: 101

Carbohydrates: 3.1g

Protein: 2.1g

Fat: 0.6g

Sugar: 0.6g

Sodium: 14mg

Fiber: 1.2g

Ultra-Spicy Almonds

Preparation time: 15 minutes

Cooking time: 2 hours & 30 minutes

Servings: 32

Ingredients

- 2½ tablespoons coconut oil

- cups of raw almonds

- garlic cloves, minced

- 1 teaspoon smoked paprika

- 2 teaspoons red chili powder

- 1 teaspoon ground cumin

- 1 teaspoon onion powder

- Salt

- ground black pepper

Directions:

1   Set a slow cooker on high and preheat for about 25 minutes.

2   Add all Ingredients and stir to combine.

3   Cook on low, uncovered, for about 2 hours, stirring occasionally.

4   Then, in high and cook, uncovered, within 30 minutes.

5   Cool before serving.

Nutrition:

Calories: 80

Carbohydrates: 2.9g

Protein: 2.6g

Fat: 7.1g

Sugar: 0.6g

Sodium: 6mg

Fiber: 1.6g

Desserts

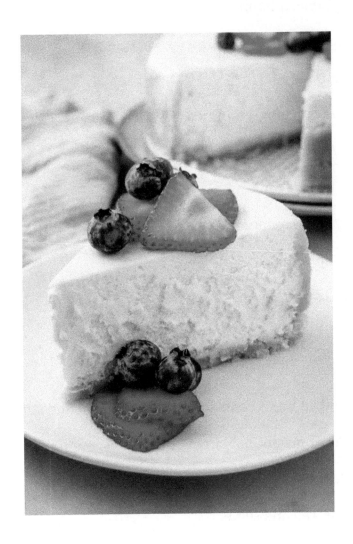

Rice Pudding

Preparation Time: 10 minutes

Cooking Time: 4 hours

Servings: 6

Ingredients:

- 3/4 cup long-grain rice

- 3/4 cup sugar

- 3 cups of milk

- 1/2 tsp cinnamon

- 1 tsp vanilla

- 2 tbsp butter

- 1/4 tsp salt

Directions:

1. Add all ingredients into the cooking pot and stir well.

2. Cover instant pot aura with lid.

3. Select slow cook mode and cook on LOW for 4 hours.

4. Stir well and serve.

Nutrition: calories 276, fat 6, carbs 13, protein 14

Delicious Bread Pudding

Preparation Time: 10 minutes

Cooking time: 4 hours

Servings: 8

Ingredients:

- 5 eggs

- 8 cups of bread cubes

- 1 tbsp vanilla

- 4 cups of milk

- 3/4 cup maple syrup

- 1 tbsp cinnamon

Directions:

1. In a large bowl, whisk together eggs, sugar, cinnamon, vanilla, and milk.

2. Add bread cubes into the cooking pot.

3. Pour egg mixture on top of bread cubes and let sit for 15 minutes.

4. Cover instant pot aura with lid.

5. Select slow cook mode and cook on LOW for 4 hours.

6. Serve and enjoy.

Nutritional values per serving: calories 153, fat 4.74, carbs 23.26, protein 5.27

Lightning Source UK Ltd.
Milton Keynes UK
UKHW020645010621
384724UK00004B/16

9 781802 971132